ESSENTIALS OF ORTHOPEDIC TECHNIQUES

First edition. January 28, 2024.

ISBN: 979-8224976676

Written by yingxiong feng.

Table of Contents

Essentials of Orthopedic Techniques

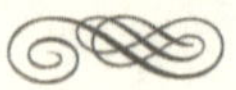

By Yingxiong Feng

ABOUT THE AUTHOR:

The author is a TCM doctor, teacher and Buddhist practitioner. He has published 20 books in Buddhism, culture and health.

"Every Person Is Their Own Best Doctor - Chinese Traditional Medicine In Practice" is one of the author's works on TCM clinical practice that also serves as an introduction to TCM.

Praised by many as "The best TCM doctor in New York Chinatown", "Loved by all his patients", "Patients' last hope".

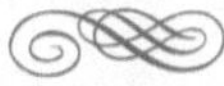

COPYRIGHT

Catalog

Injury leading to stupor or unconsciousness
Injury causing vomiting
Injury resulting in thirst
Injury with constipation

Introduction

Traditional Chinese bone-setting is a conventional Chinese medical practice primarily used for treating fractures, dislocations, muscle and ligament injuries. This method combines the holistic concepts of traditional Chinese medicine with unique therapeutic techniques, which mainly include:

Manual Reduction: This technique involves manually adjusting dislocated or fractured parts to their correct anatomical positions. This method requires the practitioner to have profound knowledge in anatomy and traditional Chinese medicine theory, as well as extensive clinical experience.

Application or Ingestion of Chinese Herbal Medicine: Chinese herbal medicines are used to promote wound healing, reduce inflammation and pain, and stimulate blood circulation to dissipate blood stasis. Topically applied medicines usually consist of herbal mixtures applied directly to the injured area, while oral medicines are ingested to achieve a systemic treatment effect.

Tui Na and Massage: This involves specific massage techniques aimed at improving local blood circulation, facilitating the recovery of muscles and ligaments, and reducing pain and stiffness.

Acupuncture: Acupuncture is used to regulate the balance of Qi (energy) and blood within the body, alleviate pain, and promote the self-healing of injured areas.

Functional Exercise: During the recovery phase, specific functional exercises or physical therapy may be recommended to strengthen muscle power and increase the flexibility and stability of joints.

The principle of treatment in traditional Chinese bone-setting is holistic regulation. It focuses not only on the local treatment of the wound but also considers the overall physical condition and constitution of the patient. It is important to emphasize that traditional Chinese bone-setting should be performed by experienced professionals, especially in the case of complex fractures and dislocations, where careful handling is essential. In some instances, it is also necessary to integrate modern medical techniques, such as X-ray examinations, to ensure the safety and effectiveness of the treatment.

In this book, I am going to talk about the Key Principles of Bone-Setting in in the context of traditional Chinese medicine. These are the core principles or essential techniques in traditional bone-setting or orthopedic practices in ancient China.

My discussion is mainly based on the clinical practice by Dr. Wu Qian, imperial physician in the Imperial Court of the Qing Dynasty and my translation of his "Zheng Gu Xin Fa" or Essentials Of Orthopedic Techniques.

General Discussion of Traditional Bone-setting or Manual Therapy in TCM

THE TERM "MANUAL TECHNIQUE" of "manual therapy" refers to the use of both hands to adjust the injured muscles and bones, restoring them to their original state. However, injuries vary in severity, and different hand techniques are appropriate for different cases.

The speed of recovery, as well as whether any physiological disabilities remain, largely depends on the appropriateness of the hand technique applied, whether it misses the mark, or whether it is not fully executed.

Since the skeletal structure of the body is not uniform, and the arrangement and connections of the twelve meridian sinews are all different, it is essential to have a fundamental understanding of the body's structure and recognize the specific parts involved.

In practice, when responding to a case, the skill emerges from within, the hands follow the heart, and the technique flows from the hands.

Whether it involves pulling to separate and then realign, pushing to adjust and reposition, straightening what is crooked, or completing what is missing, in cases of bone fractures—whether complete, fragmented, or slanted—and in cases of tendons being lax, taut, curled, cramped, flipped, twisted, separated, or joined, even though these lie within the flesh, they can be fully understood by hand palpation.

The application of technique, making the patient unaware of any pain, is what truly defines manual skill.

Moreover, since many injuries involve vital areas, such as the seven apertures connecting to the brain, the diaphragm close to the heart, and limbs whose injuries cause deep-seated pain, even if a person is generally strong, carelessly applied techniques can lead to severe consequences, and recovery might be hard to achieve.

This is why precision and caution are especially important. A skilled bone-setter must have both an insightful mind and adept hands, understand the condition, and skillfully apply manual techniques to be effective in treatment.

Indeed, the hands, being part of the body, possess the remarkable ability to perform subtle and versatile movements, using their own tension and relaxation, movement and stillness, quickness and slowness, lightness and heaviness, opening and closing, to address issues like blood and qi stagnation, swelling and pain in the skin and muscles, cramping and breaking of tendons and bones, as well as emotional distress.

Compared to using instruments for restrictive procedures, the difference is significant. Thus, manual technique is indeed the primary task in bone-setting.

Different Kinds of Manual Techniques

Palpation - Feeling by touch

Palpation involves using the hands to delicately feel the injured area. This can include sensing whether the bones are broken, fractured, misaligned, intact, soft, or hard, and whether the tendons are strong, flexible, twisted, straight, torn, displaced, thick, flipped, cold, or hot. It also involves assessing the superficial and deep aspects of the injury, as well as determining whether it is a new or old ailment. Initially, one feels for injuries that may have resulted from falls, sprains, or impacts, and then treatment is administered according to the diagnosis.

Reduction - Setting of bones

Reduction refers to the process of bringing together the ends of a broken bone to allow it to heal in its original position. In cases where the bones are injured from a fall, dislocated, broken into two pieces, bent or depressed, shattered and scattered, or protruding at an angle, the situation should be assessed, and the bones are gently manipulated back into place. This involves ensuring that the broken parts are reconnected, the depressed areas are lifted, the shattered parts are made whole again, and the protruding parts are smoothed out. This may be done using manual techniques, tools, or a combination of both, sequentially or concurrently, depending on the practitioner's expertise and judgment.

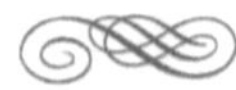

ALIGNMENT - POSITIONING

Alignment involves using one or both hands to firmly grasp and position the affected area. Depending on the severity of the condition, this might involve lifting from below upwards, pushing from outside inwards, or aligning straight or at an angle. When a bone is dislocated, it must be aligned using this technique. Prompt and correct alignment ensures that the bone will heal properly without unnecessary delay, and it is crucial to align it precisely to prevent any future issues with uneven length or misalignment.

Elevation - lifting

Elevation refers to the process of lifting a bone that has been depressed or sunken back to its original position. There are various methods for this: some use both hands to lift, others use ropes or cloths tied to a higher point for elevation, and still others elevate and then use tools to prevent the bone from sinking again. The severity and depth of the injury must be carefully assessed before treatment is applied. If a serious injury is treated too lightly, healing may not occur; conversely, if a minor injury is treated too aggressively, the original problem may be resolved but new issues may arise.

Massage Therapy

"Pressing" refers to applying downward pressure with the hands. "Rubbing" means to gently knead or massage. This method is particularly used for injuries to the skin, muscles, and tendons that are swollen, hardened, or numb, but where the bones are not broken or fractured. It's often applied in cases where a fall or a misstep causes the bone joints to misalign, leading to blocked qi (energy) and blood circulation, resulting in swelling and pain. Massage therapy is suitable in these situations. Pressing along the meridians can help to unblock stagnant qi, and rubbing the congested areas can help to disperse blood stasis and reduce swelling, thereby aiding in recovery.

Tuina Method

"Pushing" involves using the hands to push the affected area back to its original position. "Grasping" means using one or both hands to firmly grasp the affected area, applying pressure as appropriate, either gently or firmly, to slowly restore it to its proper place. If swelling and pain have subsided and the injury appears healed, but there are still issues like tight tendons making movement difficult, or if the tendons are overstretched affecting mobility, or if there are slight misalignments in the bone joints, these issues indicate that although the injury seems healed, the flow of qi (energy) and blood is not yet smooth. In such cases, methods like alignment, positioning, or elevation are not suitable; instead, Tuina is appropriate to open and regulate the flow of energy and blood through the meridians. The human body has major and minor meridians, and through careful pushing and grasping, considering the specific conditions of deficiency or excess, methods of invigorating or regulating can be applied, aiding in the patient's recovery.

These points summarize the eight methods. As for the balance and skill required in practice, the ability to apply these with a combination of divine insight and clear understanding depends on the practitioner."

General Discussion on Instruments

When injuries from falls are treated with manual methods, there may be limitations in fully achieving the desired results, leading to situations where the treatment feels ineffective. Therefore, it cannot be said that the medical approach is comprehensive. Considering the body's upper and lower parts, and its front and sides, instruments are designed to correct these aspects, aiding where manual techniques fall short. They are used in the hope of rejoining separated parts, straightening the slanted, leveling the elevated, and raising the sunken. Thus, critical conditions can be turned to safety, and severe injuries can be made lighter.

Furthermore, when combined with the efficacy of medicinal treatments and supplemented with proper nourishment and care, the practice of orthopedics becomes complete.

Wrapping with Cloth or Bandaging

This technique involves the use of white cloth. It is used in cases where the affected area is not suitable for other instruments and is only appropriate for wrapping with cloth. This is considered the correct method, hence the name 'wrapping with cloth.' The length and width of the cloth should be chosen based on the severity and nature of the injury.

Wooden Stick

This tool is about one and a half feet long and as round as a coin. A flat stick can also be used. It is applied to areas of injury where qi (energy) and blood have stagnated, causing pain and hardness. By gently tapping around the injured area with this stick, qi and blood circulation can be promoted, leading to dispersion of these blockages. As a result, pain gradually decreases and the hardness or swelling slowly resolves.

Method Explanation:

For head injuries where the bones are not broken and the tendons are not torn, treatment is possible even in cases of swelling and pain caused by bruising. First, use manual techniques to adjust and lift the neck, nape, and the tendons and bones. Then, wrap the head with cloth in two or three layers tightly. After that, gently tap the sole of the foot with a tapping stick to facilitate the upward and downward movement of the qi (vital energy) of the five organs. This helps to disperse the stagnant blood, preventing it from rushing towards the heart, and also prevents nausea and hiccupping, thus calming the mind and spirit.

However, if after wrapping the head and tapping the sole of the foot, there is still no sensation of pain, and the patient is unconscious and unresponsive, with a phlegm sound resembling the sawing of wood, a rigid body, drooling from the mouth, then it is a case of critical depletion of qi and blood, and is considered untreatable.

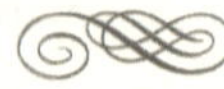

SHOULDER WRAP

A shoulder wrap involves using a piece of cured cowhide, measuring five inches in length and three inches in width, with two holes at each end. It is placed over the injured area, threaded through with cotton rope, and tightly bound. Compared to a wooden board, it feels slightly more flexible.

Method Explanation:

In cases of injuries where both shoulders are dislocated or misaligned, with fractured or protruding bones, or misaligned joints and tendons, the treatment involves having the patient lie on a bench, aligning the bone joints, and massaging and pressing the tendon structures. Cotton is used for padding against the body, and the shoulder wrap is placed over the front and back of the shoulders, tightly bound with cotton rope. Following this, a white cloth is used for additional wrapping. A supporting board, over two feet in length and three to four inches in width, is threaded with ropes at both ends and suspended, allowing the patient to lie face down without letting the shoulder bones hang down. After seven days, the condition is reevaluated. If the injuries have healed, the board can be removed; if not, it should continue to be used. Failure to follow this treatment may lead to lingering issues with the joints.

Climbing Rope

Climbing rope refers to using a rope hung from a high place, which is then climbed using both hands.

Stacking Bricks

Stacking bricks involves using six bricks, dividing them into two sets of three each, placed on the left and right, respectively, for both feet to stand on.

Application Explanation:

For cases involving injuries to the chest, abdomen, internal organs, or ribs, caused by falls, strikes, jumps, collisions, pushes, or exertions, resulting in a sunken chest, the patient is first instructed to grasp a rope with both hands and stand on bricks. Holding the patient's lower back, remove one brick from each side, encouraging the patient to straighten their body and chest out. After a short while, remove another brick from each side and ask the patient to straighten again. Repeat this three times until the patient's feet touch the ground, allowing the energy to flow and dissipate the stagnation, thereby raising the sunken area and straightening what is bent. Then, wrap the chest with a bamboo mat and tightly bind it with eight wide straps, ensuring it's not too constrictive. The patient should sleep on their back, avoid lying face down or on their side, and use a pillow under their waist to prevent shifting from side to side.

Wood Device

This device is made from fir wood, three inches wide and two inches thick, with a length extending from the waist, over the shoulders, and up by about half an inch. The outer surface is smooth, while the inner surface facing the spine is carved into a concave shape to snugly fit the spinal bones and muscles, approximately five-inch deep. Starting from one side, diagonally drill two holes at the first half inch, and similarly, two holes on the opposite side. From the second to the fifth half inch, drill one hole on each side, diagonally. Use a wide strap, threading it through the upper left hole at the first half inch, passing over the right shoulder, across the chest, diagonally towards the lower left side, around the back, and through the right hole at the same inch. Then, use another strap, threading it through the upper right hole at the first half inch, passing over the left shoulder, across the chest, diagonally towards the lower right side, around the back, and through the left hole at the same inch. Tie both straps tightly to the wood. For the third, fourth, and fifth half inch, similarly thread straps through the holes, wrapping them horizontally around the ribs and abdomen, then back through the original holes, and tie them tightly to the wood. At the fifth inch, thread the strap through the hole, wrap it around the abdomen, then tie it tightly at the back. Ensure it does not shift or move to be effective on the affected area. Before using this wood, pad it with soft cotton and silk against the body to prevent pain.

Method of Application Explanation:

For those who have suffered a fall or blow to the spine, resulting in cracked and protruding vertebrae, the patient often exhibits a hunched back and difficulty in looking upwards. The appropriate treatment involves having the patient lie face down. Then, another person stands on the patient's shoulders with their feet. The practitioner should then treat the cracked and protruding area, judging whether to apply light or heavy pressure, and whether to use techniques such as aligning, grabbing, pressing, or kneading, to facilitate the closure of the crack. Afterwards, use the wooden device as previously described to press down on the area.

Waist Column

The waist column is made of four pieces of fir wood, fashioned in the shape of a carrying pole, each one inch wide and half an inch thick. The length of each piece is determined by the size of the affected area. Holes are drilled on the side of each piece, and they are strung together with a rope.

Method of Use Explanation:

For general waist injuries such as sprains, strains, or misalignments, standard treatment methods are used. However, in cases where the spinal joints are injured, the back muscles are torn, or the tendons are abnormally bent and causing a stooped posture, vinegar mixed with pain-relieving herbs is applied on the waist columns. These columns are then arranged along both sides of the spine, ensuring they are aligned properly. Next, moxa (made from mugwort) is used to create a thin mat, which is placed over the columns to protect against cold and wind. A wide and long cloth band is then wrapped around the abdomen and tied tightly to secure everything in place. Internal medication is also administered to aid the healing process.

Bamboo Mat

This refers to the cooling bamboo mats commonly used in the summer. It should be cut according to the size and length required for the injured area.

Method of Use Explanation:

For any limb with a fracture, first set the bone using manual methods. Then, wrap the area with cloth, and subsequently encircle it with the bamboo mat over the cloth. Secure it tightly to ensure that the bone alignment remains uniform without any misalignment or displacement. This is a universally applied method in such cases.

Cedar Lattice

The cedar lattice is also a device for applying pressure. It is custom-made from cedar wood according to the length, width, curvature, and shape of the injured area, whether it's straight, curved, convex, or concave. The number of slats should be carefully chosen and arranged in a clear order to avoid confusion. Then, a hole is drilled at each end of every slat, and they are connected with a rope. It resembles a lattice, hence the name. However, it is arranged more sparsely than a bamboo mat, not as closely packed.

Usage Explanation:

The cedar lattice is used to wrap around the outside of the bamboo mat. The ropes threaded through it are tied securely, and additional ropes are added to the lattice for wrapping, ensuring firmness and straightness, preventing the bones from shifting or dislocating. This is particularly important at the joints where bones are long and prone to movement. If only a bamboo mat is used, it might not provide sufficient rigidity, hence the necessity of adding the cedar lattice for additional support. This ensures a firm and aligned healing of the bone.

Embrace Knee

The Embrace Knee is a bamboo ring with four legs. Made of bamboo strips, the ring is slightly larger than the knee. Four more bamboo strips are tightly bound to the ring with hemp thread to form a four-legged structure. Strips of white cloth are then wrapped around the bamboo ring and its four legs. When used on the knee, it restricts movement without causing pain.

Usage and Explanation:

The kneecap covers the ends of the femur and tibia and is naturally mobile. If injured, it may not necessarily involve bone fracture but could be dislocated and protrude to the sides. Even if manually repositioned, any movement or walking can cause it to shift again. Therefore, the Embrace Knee device is used to secure it, preventing it from moving out of place again and avoiding the risk of a permanent limp. To use this method, insert the four legs of the Embrace Knee on either side of the knee. The bamboo ring then encircles and stabilizes the knee, ensuring it cannot move. Finally, wrap it tightly with a wide strip of white cloth to secure it in place.

Theoretical basis From TCM Classics

Theory For treating injuries from falls by acupuncture at various points from Huangdi Neijing - The Yellow Emperor's Innor Canon

"Suwen · Miu Ci Lun" (◇◇·◇◇◇) states:

"When a person falls or collapses, bad blood accumulates internally, causing fullness and swelling in the abdomen, and hindering movement forwards or backwards. First, administer a diuretic. This condition injures the Jueyin (◇◇) meridian of the upper body and the Shaoyin (◇◇) network of the lower body. Puncture below the inner ankle, and the blood vessel in front of the Rangu (◇◇) point to release blood. Puncture the artery on the upper part of the foot. If this is not effective, puncture each of the San Mao (San Mao" refers to the area located behind the toenail of the big toe, corresponding to the second phalangeal section of the big toe.) points to draw blood until the issue resolves. Puncture the left side for issues on the right, and the right side for issues on the left."

This passage describes a traditional Chinese medicine approach for treating internal injuries caused by falls, focusing on acupuncture techniques to release bad blood and alleviate swelling.

The above quotation discusses the concept that 'evil blood' causes illness and can be treated with acupuncture. When a person falls and sustains an injury, it can lead to internal retention of 'evil blood,' resulting in abdominal fullness and obstruction. In such cases, potent medicines should be used initially. If the injury affects the Jueyin liver meridian above and the Shaoyin kidney meridian below, acupuncture should be performed below the inner ankle, anterior to the point known as Ran Gu. If there is a blood vessel here that bleeds when pricked, it indicates the branch of the Shaoyin meridian that communicates with the Jueyin meridian. Additionally, acupuncture should be done on the dorsal artery of the foot, at the Chongyang point, which is the source point of the stomach meridian. If the condition does not improve, further acupuncture should be performed on the Dadun point located above 'San Mao' on both sides of the big toe. Blood should be drawn immediately upon needling. For contralateral needling, needle the right Dadun point for a problem on the left, and vice versa. However, when needling the dorsal artery of the foot, the Chong pulse, and the Shaoyin and Yangming meridians, only shallow needling should be performed, and excessive bleeding must be avoided.

"Lingshu Jing" (◇◇◇-◇◇◇◇**The Spiritual Pivot) - 'Chapter on Cold and Heat Diseases' states:**

"When the body is injured, resulting in excessive bleeding, or when affected by a stroke of cold, or if there has been a fall, leading to weakness and a lack of control in the limbs, this is called 'physical lethargy.' To treat this, one should acupuncture the point three cun (a traditional Chinese unit of measurement) below the navel, at the intersection of the three junctions. This intersection point, called 'San Jie Jiao,' involves the Yangming and Taiyin meridians, and the point three cun below the navel is known as 'Guan Yuan.'"

This passage describes a condition caused by physical trauma or exposure to certain environmental factors and suggests a specific acupuncture point for treatment. It reflects the holistic and meridian-based approach of traditional Chinese medicine.

This statement refers to those who have sustained injuries resulting in heavy bleeding, or those who have been struck by wind-cold, which is related to tetanus. Alternatively, it could be due to a fall. Even without external bleeding, if there is weakness and a lack of control in the limbs, these are all categorized as 'physical lethargy.' The point called 'Guan Yuan' is an acupuncture point on the Ren meridian, and also a junction where the foot Yangming and Taiyin meridians meet, hence it is referred to as the intersection of three junctions.

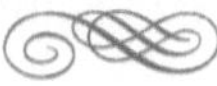

THE 'LING SHU JING'(◈◈◈-◈◈◈) **in the chapter on syncope disorders states:**

"For headaches that should not be treated with acupuncture, if they are caused by a blow or fall resulting in internal pooling of 'bad blood' and the pain is persistent, it is appropriate to perform acupuncture at nearby points, but not at distant points."

This excerpt implies that in cases of headache due to trauma with suspected internal bleeding or hematoma, acupuncture treatment should be localized and not done on points far from the site of injury. This is a specific guideline within the broader context of traditional Chinese medical practice."

The text states that for headaches caused by internal 'bad blood,' one should not perform acupuncture on the points typically used for headaches. Usually, headaches are treated by releasing qi at certain points, which can alleviate the pain. However, if the headache is due to a blow or fall causing internal 'bad blood,' then using these points to release qi would be treating a blood disorder with qi therapy, which is not advisable. Therefore, these points should not be used in such cases. If the pain from a blow or fall is persistent, even though acupuncture might be used, it should only be applied to the sides near the injured area to release the internal 'bad blood.' Relying on distant points as typically used for treating headaches according to the meridians should not be done in these cases.

This excerpt implies that in cases of headache due to trauma with suspected internal bleeding or hematoma, acupuncture treatment should be localized and not done on points far from the site of injury.

This excerpt underlines a specific principle in traditional Chinese medicine: the treatment strategy must be adapted according to the underlying cause of the symptoms. In this case, when a headache is due to traumatic injury with suspected internal bleeding, the usual acupuncture points for headache are not suitable, and a more localized treatment is recommended.

Theory For treating Bad Blood and liver injury caused by anger as the result of an accident

THE "LING SHU JING (The Spiritual Pivot), Chapter on the Forms of Diseases Caused by Pathogenic Qi in the Organs and Viscera," says:

"If there has been a fall or a similar accident, resulting in internal 'bad blood,' and if there is an occurrence of great anger causing the qi to rise and not descend, accumulating under the ribs, then the liver is injured."

This passage describes a situation in traditional Chinese medicine where physical trauma (resulting in internal 'bad blood') combined with emotional disturbance (specifically, intense anger) can lead to a pathological condition affecting the liver. The rising and non-descending qi, especially when it accumulates under the ribs, is indicative of liver injury according to this medical tradition.

If a person falls, resulting in internal (bad) blood retention, and then experiences intense anger, injuring the liver, causing the qi to rise and not descend, then the internally retained blood and the stagnant qi together accumulate under the ribs, injuring the liver. The appropriate method is first to guide out the anger qi, preventing it from accumulating in the liver, thereby avoiding liver injury. Subsequently, administer a medicinal decoction to break up the bad blood, thus eliminating any retained blood under the ribs.

This passage explains a traditional Chinese medical approach to treating a condition where physical trauma (leading to blood retention) and emotional disturbance (intense anger affecting the liver) coexist. The treatment strategy involves first addressing the emotional component (the anger qi) to prevent further liver damage, followed by administering medicinal treatments to dispel the retained blood, which is seen as a cause of the physical ailment.

The same chapter also states, "If one suffers a fall, but continues to have sex while drunk, and then sweats taking a shower after that, it results in spleen injury."

Suffering a fall leads to external bodily injury. For instance, if one has sexual intercourse after drinking, or sweats and carelessly exposes oneself to the wind, pathogenic factors invade the skin and internal body, causing internal injury. These are factors that lead to spleen injury.

This sentence describes a scenario in traditional Chinese medicine where a combination of physical trauma (such as falling while intoxicated) and exposure to certain environmental conditions (like sweating in the wind) is believed to lead to an injury of the spleen. The spleen, in this context, is understood not just in the anatomical sense but as an organ system with specific functions and attributes according to traditional Chinese medical theory.

The Suwen (Basic Questions) chapter on 'Pulse Essentials and Subtleties' states:

"If the liver pulse is firm and long, and the color is not blue, it indicates a condition of sinking or palpitations, due to blood stagnating below the ribs, causing panting and counterflow.'"

This means that the liver pulse has both firmness and softness, and the diseases also vary accordingly. When the liver pulse beats under the hand, being both firm and long, and its color is not blue, the condition is likely to be sinking or palpitations, due to blood accumulating under the ribs, causing unceasing panting and counterflow. This is because the Jueyin (Liver) meridian spreads across the ribs and follows up to the throat; its branches, furthermore, pass from the liver through the diaphragm to the lungs. Now, when blood accumulates under the ribs, the congested blood sends its qi (vital energy) upwards, suffocating the lungs, thus causing panting and counterflow.

This passage elaborates on the diagnosis of liver-related conditions in traditional Chinese medicine, focusing on the qualities of the liver pulse and their relationship to symptoms and the flow of energy (qi) within the body. The description highlights the interconnectedness of different organs and meridians (energy pathways) in Chinese medical theory, particularly how issues in the liver can affect lung function and lead to respiratory symptoms.

This passage from a classic Chinese medical text describes the diagnosis of a specific liver condition through pulse examination. In traditional Chinese medicine, the qualities of the pulse (such as firmness and length) are closely observed to determine the state of internal organs. Here, a firm and long liver pulse, without a bluish color, is associated with blood stagnation under the ribs, which in turn leads to symptoms like panting and a kind of reverse or abnormal flow of energy or breath (counterflow).

Theoretical Basis From Jin Gui Yao Lue

"THE 'JIN GUI YAO LUE' (Essential Prescriptions of the Golden Coffer) states:

"If the pulse at the 'cun' position (wrist) is floating, faint, and rough, it indicates blood loss. If there is sweating, or even if there is no sweating, and the person has sores or has been injured by a knife or an axe, it is due to loss of blood."

According to the classic, "Those who lose blood do not sweat, and those who lose sweat do not bleed. Both conditions are characterized by a pulse that is floating, faint, and rough. Observing such symptoms indicates signs of exhaustion and a lack of sweating, which are indicative of blood loss. Therefore, it is evident that there are signs of blood loss due to injuries from metal or from a fall."

This passage describes a specific diagnostic observation from traditional Chinese medicine, focusing on the characteristics of the pulse at the wrist and their implications regarding the patient's condition, particularly in relation to blood loss and its various possible causes.

I explain a bit more on this statement. When the liver pulse is firm but the color remains unchanged, it is likely due to a fall or a similar incident. If the flesh is not broken, then the bad blood must have accumulated under the ribs, also causing nausea and vomiting. According to the classics, one should treat this by bleeding points such as 'Ran Gu' on the foot or 'San Mao', or by drinking a medicinal decoction that disperses the bad blood, which should lead to recovery. If the pulse is floating, faint, and rough, it indicates excessive blood loss. According to the classics, one should apply moxibustion to the 'San Jie Jiao' and 'Guan Yuan' acupoints, or drink a tonic that greatly replenishes qi and blood to regulate the condition, and then the illness should be resolved.

Dimensions of Bones in the "Ling Shu Jing" (The Spiritual Pivot)

Head Measurement

FROM THE HAIRLINE AT the back of the neck to the back, the bone length is two and a half inches. (This refers to the distance from the rear hairline to the third cervical vertebra, also known as the large vertebra.)

Note on Head Measurement Method:

Please first note that the measurement "inch" in TCM is somewhat different from the actual length in western standards.

Measure from the front hairline to the rear hairline, which should be one foot and two inches. If the hairline is not clear, take the midpoint of the eyebrows, measure straight up to the back to the large vertebra, which should be one foot and eight inches; this is considered the direct inch. The horizontal inch method: measure from the inner corner of the eye to the outer corner, this is one inch. The head's horizontal and direct inch measurements are based on this method.

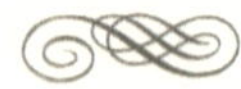

Chest and Abdomen Measurement

FROM THE ADAM'S APPLE down to the middle of the suprasternal notch, the length is four inches. (This refers to the depression above the large bone, precisely at the notch or the location of the Tian Tu acupoint.) From below the suprasternal notch to the midpoint of the xiphoid process is nine inches long.

The circumference of the chest is four feet and five inches.

The distance between the two nipples is nine and a half inches. (The standard measurement should be eight inches.)

From the middle down to the Tianshu point, the length is eight inches. (Tianshu is the name of an acupoint in the Stomach Meridian, located beside the navel; this refers to the level of the navel.)

From the Tianshu point down to the horizontal bone, the length is six and a half inches, and the horizontal bone itself is six and a half inches long. (The horizontal bone referred to here is the bone just below the hairline of the lower abdomen.)

Note: These ancient measurements, when compared with modern acupoint measurement methods, often show inconsistencies. It is advisable to follow the later methods for measuring the back and abdomen.

The distance between the two hips is six and a half inches. (This measurement is taken at the midpoint between the thighs, at the location where the two ends of the horizontal bone meet, commonly referred to as the 'hip seam').

Note: Method for measuring the chest and abdomen: For vertical measurements, the midpoint line is used. Starting from the center of the suprasternal notch (Quepen Middle, Tian Tu acupoint), up to the upper border of the manubrium (Qi Bone, Zhong Ting acupoint), the measurement is eight inches and four parts (fen). From the lower border of the manubrium to the center of the navel (Qi Bone down to the Navel Center), the measurement is eight inches. From below the navel to the pubic symphysis (Mao Jie Qu Bone acupoint), the measurement is five inches. For horizontal measurements, the distance between the two nipples is used, measured as eight inches. Both the horizontal and vertical measurements of the chest and abdomen are based on this method.

Back Measurement

FROM THE LUMBAR VERTEBRAE down to the tailbone, spanning twenty-one sections, the length is three feet. (The lumbar vertebrae are the spinal bones. The spine is small on the outside but large on the inside, which enables humans to bear heavy loads due to the size of these bones. There are twenty-four spinal segments in total, but when it mentions twenty-one here, it excludes the three cervical vertebrae in the neck.) Waist circumference is four feet and two inches.

Note on Measuring the Back:

From the large vertebra (Da Zhui) to the tailbone, the total length is measured as three feet. The upper seven segments are each one and four-tenths of an inch, totaling nine inches and eight-tenths of an inch; the middle seven segments are each one and six-tenths of an inch, totaling eleven inches and two-tenths of an inch; the fourteenth segment is level with the navel, and the lower seven segments are each one and two-tenths of an inch, totaling eight inches and eight-tenths of an inch. The total is twenty-nine inches and nine-tenths of an inch, slightly less than three feet, with a small remainder. This is the method for measuring the length vertically. For measuring horizontally, use the middle finger and follow the same method as for measuring the body.

The spinal column is one inch wide internally. In acupuncture, when it says "the second line beside the spine is one and a half inches, the third line is three inches," these measurements are taken in addition to the one inch of the spine itself. Thus, in the second line, the total measurement is two inches, and in the third line, it is three and a half inches.

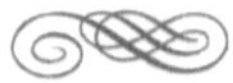

Side of the Body

- From the column bone (neck root bone) downwards to the armpit (where it becomes invisible), the length is four inches.

● From below the armpit to the end of the ribs (Ji Xie, or lower ribs), the length is one foot and two inches.

● From the end of the ribs down to the hip pivot (Bi Shu), the length is six inches. (The thigh is called "Gu," the upper part of the thigh is "Bi Jian," and the area where the two bones of the hip meet is called "Bi Shu," located at the Huan Tiao acupoint of the foot Shaoyang.)

● From the hip pivot down to the middle of the knee, the length is one foot and nine inches.

● From the upper edge of the horizontal bone down to the upper edge of the inner auxiliary bone, the length is one foot and eight inches. (The edge of the bone is called "Lian," and the bones beside the knee that protrude are called auxiliary bones, with the inner one being the inner auxiliary and the outer one being the outer auxiliary.)

● From the upper edge to the lower edge of the inner auxiliary, the length is three and a half inches. (The upper and lower edges can be felt.)

● From the lower edge of the inner auxiliary down to the ankle, the length is one foot and two inches.

● From below the inner ankle to the ground, the length is three inches.

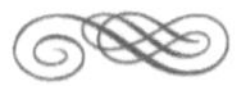

Measurement of the Limbs

● From the shoulder to the elbow, the length is one foot and seven inches.

● From the elbow to the wrist, the length is one foot and two and a half inches. (The joint in the middle of the arm is called the elbow.)

● From the wrist to the base joint of the middle finger, the length is four inches. (The joint where the arm and hand meet is called the wrist.)

● From the base joint to the tip of the finger, the length is four and a half inches. (The joint near the end of the finger is called the base joint.)

● From below the knee to the outer ankle, the length is one foot and six inches.

● From below the knee to the tarsal joint, the length is one foot and two inches. (The bend of the leg is referred to as the knee, and the tarsal refers to the top of the foot. The knee is at the front, and the calf is at the back. The tarsal joint refers to the area where the two ankles, front and back of the shin, and foot intersect.)

● From the tarsal joint down to the ground, the length is three inches.

● From the outer ankle down to the ground, the length is one inch.

- The foot is one foot and two inches long and four and a half inches wide.

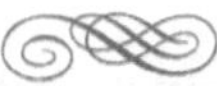

NOTE:

The measurements of bones are from the "Bone Measurements Chapter" of the "Ling Shu Jing" (Spiritual Pivot), discussing the lengths of bones in ancient units. However, it's mentioned that these measurements can vary, with larger bones possibly exceeding these numbers and smaller ones falling short. This is just a general guideline. The method of measuring the entire body and limbs is based on using the middle finger as a standard unit of measurement.

Discussion on Treatment of Bone Injuries

Head and Face

Bregma Bone

"Bregma" refers to the top of the head. In men, the bregma has a trident-shaped suture, while in women, it has a cross-shaped suture. Also known as the "Heavenly Spirit Cover," it is located at the highest point on the head, enclosing the brain like a cover, governing the entire body. In cases of sudden injury due to a fall or impact, if a person suddenly dies, the body becomes rigid, there are breathing sounds from the nose and mouth, the eyes are closed, the face turns a clay-like color, and there is a warm, throbbing sensation at the chest, then this condition is treatable. One must not abruptly lift or seat the injured person upright, as this may cause the disturbed qi to rush upwards, potentially escaping through the injury site or the seven orifices, endangering their life. Instead, it is appropriate to have them lie on their side with knees bent. First, apply a mixture of high vinegar and mixed-yuan ointment to the top of the head to alleviate pain, reduce swelling, invigorate blood circulation, and draw out toxins. Then, light a piece of herbal paper to create smoke, and let this smoke enter the mouth and nose. If available, burn coal and quench it in vinegar to produce hot vapors to fumigate the mouth and nose. If coal is not available, burning and quenching iron can also work. This is done to stimulate and harmonize the blood and qi of the five organs. Once the person starts to groan or make sounds, administer a warm mixture of child's urine with eight-li powder. This can help restore the flow of qi and bring back yang energy. Additionally, use hand techniques to massage and press the heart, chest, ribs, underarms, abdomen, and gently lift the inner wrist, frequently rubbing these areas. This includes the area behind the palm, and the cun, guan, and chi points where the pulse is measured.

In cases of concussion or impact injury, if the muscles and veins become rigid, frequent massage can help restore the heart's blood flow and ensure the vitality channel (life vein) is unblocked, leading to revival. Regularly take Zheng Gu Zi Jin Dan (Correct Bone Purple Gold Pill), and externally apply San Yu He Hang Tang (Disperse Stasis and Harmonize Injury Decoction) to wash off the previously applied Mixed Yuan Ointment before reapplying it. After taking the pill, if the stool appears black and dry, it indicates that there is stagnant blood in the gastrointestinal tract. For those who experience deafness, they should take a modified version of Su Zi Tao Ren Tang (Perilla Seed and Peach Kernel Decoction) to dispel the stagnant blood, strengthen the spleen and stomach, and nourish the spirit, while also using Dao Qi Tong Yu Ding (Qi-Guiding and Stasis-Removing Pellet) in the ears. Dietary recommendations include plain congee, soup, and drinks. It is advisable to avoid anger, greasy foods, and wheat-based products.

The patient should rest in a clean, quiet room, free from noise and disturbance. In cases where the injury is severe and the patient has passed away, wrap the head in a white cloth, gently tap the center of the foot with a wooden stick, then straighten the hair to properly align the neck bones and relax the tendons. Apply Mixed Yuan Ointment externally and administer Zi Jin Dan (Purple Gold Pill) internally. If the injury is due to a fall from a horse or carriage, causing damage to the top of the head, the injury often occurs more on the left side than the right, likely due to the convenience of using the right hand. The treatment method is the same as for concussive injuries. If the skull is collapsed, causing disturbance to the brain marrow, bleeding from the seven orifices, rigid convulsions, and complete unconsciousness, then it is considered untreatable.

For methods of treatment, including prescription of herbal formulas, pills, herbs used in moxibustion and ironing methods, plasters for applying on wounds, and herbal decoctions for washing wounds, as well as methods of preparation, please refer to the Chinese version of this book.

The medicines such as "Zheng Gu Zijin Dan" (Bone-setting Purple Gold Pill), "Hun Yuan Gao" (Mixed Origin Ointment), "San Yu He Shang Tang" (Bruise and Injury Harmonizing Decoction), "Hai Tong Pi Tang" (Sea Buckthorn Bark Decoction), and "Wan Ling Gao" (Myriad Spirit Ointment) are all commonly used and experienced prescriptions in the Imperial Court. Therefore, they are frequently referenced for the various conditions described above and below. In cases of injuries from falls or trauma that are also complicated by other illnesses, the treatment is not limited to these few medicines.

Please email isherhope@gmail.com for more information.

The Fontanel

The fontanelle, in infants, is the unjoined part of the skull on the top of the head, which is soft and pulsating, known as the fontanel. In cases of falls or strikes causing injury, if the bone sutures are cracked but the brain and tendons are not yet severely affected, symptoms may include a shiny swelling of the head and neck, facial puffiness, swollen eyes, enlarged nose, flipped lips, stiff tongue, drowsiness, and lethargy. The flesh may be swollen but without skin breakage and bleeding. The appropriate treatment is to sit the patient upright and apply a mixture of onion juice and Ding Tong San (a pain-relieving powder) on the injured area. Then, place a piece of furry paper soaked in vinegar on top of the medicine, and use a heated iron to warm the paper until the injured area feels hot and painful and the child makes a sound. Remove the medicine and apply Wan Ling Ointment, changing it every three days.

Once the pain subsides and the appetite returns, the ointment should be removed and the injury washed with He Hang Tang (Harmonizing Injury Soup), which helps eliminate wind, reduce swelling, activate blood circulation, and regulate qi (energy). In cases where the flesh is broken and bleeding, use horse dung ash to stop the bleeding first. Then apply the moxibustion method with elm bark, and take internally Ren Shen Zi Jin Dan (Ginseng Purple Gold Pill) to strengthen the spleen and stomach, boost vital energy, quench thirst, generate body fluids, improve vitality, strengthen the body, and ensure the harmonious flow of tendons and blood. Avoid irritants and spicy food, wear a soft, drawstring hat to protect from wind and cold, and stay indoors. If the flesh is severely broken, bleeding continues, bones are sunken, tendons are inverted, brain damage is likely, limbs are weak with rigid tendons, and there is no sound of breath, the condition is critical and difficult to treat. If the wound is exposed to cold wind, it is untreatable.

Shan Jiao Bone

The "Shan Jiao Bone" refers to the bones on both sides of the top of the head. In cases of injury due to falls or blows where the skin is not broken, regardless of whether it's on the left or right side, if there is purple swelling, hardness, blood stasis, concentrated pain, or symptoms like unconsciousness, closed eyes, body weakness preventing standing up, shortness of breath, inability to speak, internal restlessness, shortness of breath while lying down, and reduced food and drink intake, it's appropriate to take Zheng Gu Zi Jin Dan (Rectify Bones Purple Gold Pill) internally and apply moxibustion and ironing treatment similar to that used for injuries to the fontanel bone.

If there is flesh broken and continuous bleeding, first use horse dung ash to stop the bleeding, then cover the wound with elm bark and apply moxibustion with Ai He Ding Tong San (Mugwort Harmonizing Pain Powder). In cases of severe injury, take Ren Shen Zi Jin Dan (Ginseng Purple Gold Pill) first, then follow the aforementioned treatment. If the injury is extremely severe and leads to tetanus, it is untreatable.

Ling Yun Bone

The "Ling Yun Bone" is located below the front hairline, at the center of the forehead bone. The bones above the two eyebrows are commonly known as the "Left Tian Xian Bone" and the "Right Tian Gui Bone," which are the two frontal angles. In cases of injury from falls or blows resulting in broken skin, swelling of the face, or internal bruising that leads to vomiting of blood, symptoms such as weakness and dizziness, unconsciousness, body weakness, dry and yellowish complexion, generalized edema, irritability and thirst, chest and diaphragm pain, poor appetite, and reduced food and drink intake, one should first take Shu Xue Wan (Blood Dispersing Pills). Then, use Wu Jia Pi Tang (Five Bark Decoction) to fumigate and wash the affected area, and apply Wu Long Gao (Black Dragon Ointment) to stabilize pain and reduce swelling.

Jing Ming Bone

The "Jing Ming Bone" refers to the bones surrounding the eye socket. The bone above is known as the eyebrow ridge bone, and the bone below is connected to the upper jaw. In cases of injury from falls or impacts that result in bleeding over the face, apply a medicinal paste for cut wounds; for painful, bruised areas, apply Hun Yuan Gao (Mixed Origin Ointment). If the bones are damaged, take internally Ba Li San (Eight-Tenths Powder), and avoid raw, cold, or stimulating foods. Be aware that eating pork head meat can cause a flare-up, with recovery typically taking up to a month.

For injuries to the eye socket where the pupil remains intact, treatment is possible.

Cheekbones

The "Two Cheekbones" refer to the prominent bones on each side of the face. In cases of injury from falls or impacts, if there is swelling, hardness, and pain in the cheekbones, tightness in the jaw, difficulty in chewing, bleeding from the nostrils, and flipping of the lips, one should take Zheng Gu Zi Jin Dan (Correct Bone Purple Gold Pill) internally. Externally, use a decoction of Sea Tongue Bark for fumigation and washing, and rinse the mouth with Bi Ba San. Rest in a warm place, avoiding cold.

Nasal Bone

The bone forming the bridge of the nose is called the "Nasal Bridge Bone," extending down to the end of the nose, known as "Zhun Tou." Injuries causing indentations in the two nostrils are treatable, and bleeding is not a concern. If the nasal bridge bone is indented, use Dang Gui (Angelica) ointment for application. If the two nostrils are injured due to a fall, resulting in open wounds, or if they are cut open by a metal blade, apply a wound-sealing medicine to the injured area. Externally, use an anti-inflammatory and pain-relieving powder to reduce swelling. If the nose is dislodged due to injury, a reattachment procedure is used.

Zhong Xue Tang

Zhong Xue Tang refers to the delicate, hollow area inside the nose. In cases where an injury from a fall or blow causes incessant bleeding and loss of consciousness, it is appropriate to plug the nostrils with a specially formulated medicinal paste, "Bi Zhi Dan," and then douse the head with freshly drawn cold water. If the person appears weak, administer Ren Shen Zi Jin Dan (Ginseng and Purple Gold Pill) for internal weakness. If there is blood stasis, give them a decoction of Su Zi (Perilla Seed) and Tao Ren (Peach Kernel). If, after treatment, the bleeding continues, there is no intake of food or drink, and the person shows signs of extreme weakness, closed eyes, and a yellow complexion, death is likely within eight days. However, injuries to the nasal bridge bone itself are generally not a cause for concern.

Mouth and lips

◇◇, which refers to the mouth and lips, is the orifice responsible for speech and eating. In the event of an injury to the upper lip, such as a tear or laceration caused by a fall or a strike, use a small strip of silk to bind from the back of the head to the front, securing it in place. First, stitch the wound with a thread spun from mulberry bark, then apply a sealing medicine to the area. After that, cover the sealing medicine with a blood-stopping ointment to prevent it from opening or falling off, and avoid speaking. If the lower lip is similarly injured and torn, use a strip of silk to bind from under the chin, and treat it using the same method as for the upper lip.

Yu Tang

◈◈, located inside the mouth at the upper part, also known as 'the upper jaw', corresponds to the uvula. If injured on either side, it typically results in swelling and pain. However, if the injury is at the central part of the uvula, it can affect the nasal turbinates (commonly known as 'nasal hair') or re-injure the uvula ('Yu Tang' in common parlance), leading to continuous bleeding, swelling of the nose and eyes, a bruised and purple face, fatigue, dizziness, weakness in the limbs, and pain extending to the brain. If the injury extends to the epiglottis and the upper transverse bone, mild cases recover easily, but severe cases may result in the inability to speak. If the pain reaches the heart and diaphragm, it can cause severe unconsciousness.

In urgent cases, apply borneol and grease powder on paper and place it on the injured area to stop bleeding. Internally administer Zheng Gu Zijin Dan to disperse stasis, relieve pain, regulate qi, strengthen the spleen, calm the mind, and stabilize the will. Additionally, use a decoction made from crab roe and dragon's blood resin to rinse the mouth two to three dozen times a day. If there is discomfort in breathing and reduced food intake, daily consume persimmon frost, jade dew frost, milk skin, milk cakes, milk crisp oil, and roasted millet flour to cool and moisten the body for recovery.

The Lower Jawbone

The "Di Ge Bone," also known as the mandible or commonly referred to as the lower jawbone, is where the two sides of the jaw meet and is responsible for supporting the teeth. In cases of injury due to falls or blows, symptoms may include swelling and pain in the cheeks and lips, trembling and weakness in the jaw, difficulty eating and drinking, closed eyes, faintness of spirit, restlessness, weak breathing, and a soft body.

Treatment involves wrapping and tying the jaw with cloth and securing it at the top of the head. Internally, administer Da Shen Xiao Huo Luo Dan to reduce stasis, relieve pain, harmonize blood, regulate qi, and strengthen the spleen. Additionally, use Ren Shen Zi Jin Dan for absorption, apply Gu Chi San to strengthen the teeth, and rinse the mouth with Bi Bo San to alleviate swelling and pain at the root of the teeth. Externally, apply Wan Ling Ointment. It is advised to avoid exposure to wind, cold, and cold objects, and to refrain from emotional disturbances.

Teeth

Teeth, which grow from the gums in the mouth, are commonly known as "ya" in Chinese. They are categorized into incisors, canines, molars, and wisdom teeth (the teeth at the extreme ends of the upper and lower jaws). In cases where teeth are knocked out or lost due to falls, blows, or accidents, "Bu Gu San" (Bone Repair Powder) should be applied to the area, along with "Feng Kou Yao" (Seal Mouth Medicine). Internally, a blood-breaking medicine should be taken to alleviate pain. This medication should be prepared with water, not alcohol, as this method has proven to be quite effective.

If a tooth is broken or injured but not displaced, "Fu Rong Gao" (Hibiscus Paste) should be applied. In cases where a tooth is loose, burn Ji Li (Tribulus Terrestris) roots to ash and use the ash regularly to stabilize the tooth; it will become firm. Alternatively, "Gu Chi San" (Strengthen Teeth Powder) can also be used frequently for a similar effect.

Fu Sang Bone

The "Fu Sang Bone" refers to the areas adjacent to the two frontal bones, near the sunken areas inside the temples. In cases of injury due to falls or impact, symptoms may include swelling, bleeding, bruising with a purplish and hard appearance, headache, tinnitus (ringing in the ears), blue marks covering the face, aversion to cold, internal heat, and dry stools. For such conditions, it is appropriate to take "Zheng Gu

Zi Jin Dan" (Correct Bone Purple Gold Pill) internally. If there is a physical break or lesion, use moxibustion or hot ironing techniques to relieve pain. For external breaks, apply "Wu Long Gao" (Black Dragon Ointment).

Yu Liang Bone

The "Yu Liang Bone" refers to the bone at the entrance of the ear. This area is located above the curved part of the cheek and below the cheekbone, acting as a clamp between the two bones. The inner part of the ear entrance connects upwards to the brain marrow and is also key to sensory clarity. In cases of bruising or impact injuries that affect the bones and flesh in this area, leading to swelling, pain, and bleeding, it is advisable to take "Zheng Gu Zi Jin Dan" (Correct Bone Purple Gold Pill) internally and wash the area with "Ba Xian Xiao Yao Tang" (Eight Immortals Free and Easy Wanderer Soup). After washing, apply "Hun Yuan Gao" (Primordial Ointment) and rest in a place away from cold. If the injury is severe and extends to the brain marrow and affects sensory clarity, resulting in unconsciousness, an inability to eat or drink, and if the person has a pre-existing condition of weak qi and blood, it is likely to be an incurable condition.

Liang Diao Bone

The "Liang Diao Bone," also known as Qu Jia (Curved Cheeks), refers to the part of the upper cheekbones that form a clamp, shaped like a ring, designed to accommodate the hooks of the lower jawbone. In cases of injury due to falls or other accidents, symptoms may include swollen ears, hardening of the cheeks, tightness in the jaw, and difficulty in chewing. The appropriate treatment involves taking "Zheng Gu Zi Jin Dan" (Correct Bone Purple Gold Pill) internally and applying "Wan Ling Gao" (Myriad Spirit Ointment) externally. It is also recommended to rest in a place away from cold.

Jia Che Bone

The "Jia Che Bone" refers to the bone of the lower jaw, commonly known as the "Yao Di" (Dental Hook), which supports all teeth and facilitates chewing. It's called "Jia Che" (Cheek Vehicle) due to its role in the movement of chewing. The end of this bone is hook-shaped and connects to the ring of the upper cheekbone (Qu Jia). Dislocations can occur due to falls or as a result of rheumatic attacks affecting the hook and ring joint. A single dislocation is called a "mistake," while a double dislocation is termed a "fall."

For treating a single dislocation, one method involves manually adjusting the non-dislocated side, holding the lower jaw with both hands, gently pulling it outward, and then pushing it inward to fit both sides back into the upper ring. Then, the jaw is secured with a cloth wrapped from the "Di Ge" (lower jawbone area) around the top of the head. Treatment includes taking "Zheng Gu Zi Jin Dan" (Correct Bone Purple Gold Pill) internally and applying "Wan Ling Gao" (Myriad Spirit Ointment) externally. Once the patient can eat and drink, the cloth is removed and only a chin support is used, tied to the top of the head, with recovery typically in two to three days. The treatment for a double dislocation follows the same method. A dislocation caused by yawning, which is usually more sudden and slippery, is not serious. Such dislocations are colloquially referred to as "hanging the lower jaw."

Hou Shan Bone

The "Hou Shan Bone" refers to the occipital bone at the back of the head. Its shape varies, resembling the Chinese characters for "◇" (pin), "◇" (shan), "◇" (chuan), or appearing round and pointed, like a crescent moon, a sprout, or a chicken egg, all of which are forms of the occipital bone. When injured, symptoms include dizziness, tinnitus, stiff neck, difficulty swallowing, difficulty eating, restlessness, and weakness in the limbs. Treatment involves taking "Zheng Gu Zi Jin Dan" (Correct Bone Purple Gold Pill) internally, applying "Wu Long Gao" (Black Dragon Ointment) externally, and washing the area with "Hai Tong Pi Tang" (Cassia Twig Bark Decoction) to disperse blood stasis, numbness, and alleviate pain.

In cases of severe injury to the Hou Shan Bone, such as from a high fall, with symptoms like inverted tendons, shortness of breath, phlegm making a sawing noise, drooping head, closed eyes, and wheezing, this indicates a critical condition due to wind-heat invasion and is generally untreatable. If urinary incontinence occurs, the prognosis is typically fatal. The crescent moon-shaped occipital bone is particularly prone to injury. If shaken or hit, causing the top of the skull to vibrate and the brain to twist and turn painfully, leading to unconsciousness, immediate treatment is needed. Cool water should be used to wet the hair, the jaw should be opened, and "Ba Li San" (Eight-tenths Powder) mixed with alcohol should be administered. If the person regains consciousness, feels pain, and cries, this is a sign of potential recovery. Continue treatment with "Zheng Gu Zi Jin Dan" and nourish with fried rice porridge for recovery.

Shou Tai Bone

The "Shou Tai Bone," also known as the "Wan Bone(◇◇)," is located behind the ear and connects to the "Yu Lou Bone" of the ear. In cases of injury due to falls or blows, both above and below the ear may swell. If the "Jin Bone" inside the ear is damaged, blood, pus, and fluid may be observed. External bruising around the ear can lead to painful coagulation and stiffness, causing dizziness, blurred vision, pain and swelling in the "Tai Yang" and "Fu Sang Bones" (temporal area), stiffness in the neck muscles, a floating red-purple appearance, mental fatigue, weakness in the limbs, restlessness, and reduced appetite.

Treatment involves applying "Wu Long Gao" (Black Dragon Ointment) to the injured area around the ear, using silk cotton to facilitate the flow of qi and reduce stasis with a "Tong Yu Ding" plug in the ear. Internally, "Ren Shen Zi Jin Dan" is administered to dissipate blood stasis and reduce swelling. Externally, "Ba Xian Xiao Yao Tang" is used for fumigation and washing to alleviate the swelling and pain. Consumption of hot and stimulating foods should be avoided. If there is unstoppable bleeding and no food intake for three days, it is likely that the brain marrow is affected, making the condition untreatable.

Xuan Tai Bone

The "Xuan Tai Bone," also known as the "Yu Zhu Bone (◇◇◇)," refers to the three sections of the cervical vertebrae at the back of the neck, sometimes called the "Tian Zhu Bone." There are four main types of injuries to this bone:

1. Falling from a height, causing the neck bone to be driven inward, but with some remaining mobility: Treated with the "lifting neck" method.
2. Injury from a blow, leading to an inability to raise the head: Treated with the "straightening" method.
3. Injury from a fall, causing the head to tilt to one side: Treated with the "alignment" method.
4. Injury from falling face upwards, causing either elongated tendons and displaced bones, concentrated tendons, or stiff tendons and lowered head: Treated with a combination of "pushing," "straightening," "connecting," and "aligning" methods.

When treating such injuries, the practitioner should inquire whether the injury was caused by a fall from a vehicle or horse, a fall from a high place, a severe blow, or a heavy fall. They should also ask if the patient has an appetite, if there are any injuries to the limbs, the state of their mental health, whether they can sit up and walk, if they are unconscious and not speaking, or if they are experiencing continuous pain, swelling, stiffness, or tendon swelling. For all these conditions, "Zheng Gu Zi Jin Dan" should be taken internally, "Wan Ling Gao" applied externally, and "Hai Tong Pi Tang" used for washing. Pain can be managed with moxibustion. External treatment should follow the methods detailed in the first volume.

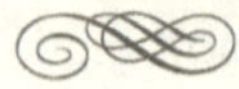

Chest and Back

COLLARBONE

The "Suo Zi Bone"(or◇◇) is the clavicle or collarbone. It lies horizontally outside the shoulder girdle, with both ends connecting to the shoulder joints. Injuries to the clavicle can occur from impacts, horseback riding, or falling while reaching for something, potentially resulting in a fracture.

To treat such an injury, the following steps are advised:

- First, press on the chest area near the injury.

- Then, gently bring the ends of the shoulder towards each other to realign the broken bone.

- Massage the fractured area to help it return to its proper position.

- Use a strap to hang the arm from the neck, ensuring that the affected area remains immobilized and does not shake.

- Internally, take "Ren Shen Zi Jin Dan" (Ginseng Purple Gold Pill) for healing.

- Apply heat to fix the pain and use "Wan Ling Gao" externally.

Following these steps, the condition should improve.

Chest Bone

Chest bone refers to the central structure of the rib cage, commonly known as the sternum. The sides of the rib cage, extending from the armpits down to the end of the ribs, are collectively known in Chinese as "Xie." The lower, smaller ribs are called "Ji Xie," commonly referred to as the "soft ribs." The term "rib" refers to each individual bone, and the collective set of ribs and sternum is known by another name.

Injuries to the sternum can vary in severity depending on whether the impact is from the front or the back, with front impacts generally being more serious. For less severe injuries, initial treatment involves specific manual therapy techniques, followed by the internal administration of "Zheng Gu Zi Jin Dan" (Correct Bone Purple Gold Pill), and external application of a pain-relief mixture made from wheat bran, along with moxibustion or heat treatment, or washing with "Hai Tong Pi Tang" (Sea Tongue Skin Soup), and applying "Wan Ling Gao." This should be effective for such cases.

If there is internal blood stasis leading to swelling, pain, and difficulty in straightening the back, treatment in the morning should include "Qing Shang Yu Xue Tang" (Clear Upper Stasis Blood Soup) and "Xiao Xia Po Xue Tang" (Disperse Lower Break Blood Soup) to address issues above and below the diaphragm, respectively, and "Shu Xue Wan" (Disperse Blood Pills) in the evening.

For long-standing injuries where the sternum is protruding, the muscles are atrophied, and there is internal pathogenic heat and blood stasis, along with feelings of fullness, tiredness, phlegm, asthma, and coughing, the prescription of "Zi Jin Dan" should be modified to reduce heat, transform phlegm, regulate qi, strengthen the spleen, nourish muscles, and stabilize breathing.

However, in cases of severe injury with internal dryness in the chest affecting the heart and lungs, symptoms like disordered qi, unconsciousness, closed eyes, vomiting of blood, hiccuping, and trembling indicate a critical condition that is beyond medical treatment.

For injuries to the ribs on both sides, the severity of the injury dictates the treatment approach. For minor injuries to the chest and ribs, medicines like "Li Dong Wan" and "San Huang Bao La Wan" are essential and should be used appropriately.

Qi Gu

The "Qi Gu (◇◇)" refers to the area where the two ends of the clavicle bones meet, located just above the manubrium, also known as the "Jiu Wei Gu" (◇◇◇Pigeon Tail Bone). This area, being close to the heart, is particularly sensitive and vulnerable to injury. Injuries here, whether due to a fall or being struck, often result in blood stasis and significant pain. In mild cases, the impact affects only the area above the diaphragm, but in severe cases, it can affect the heart, leading to symptoms like unconsciousness, closed eyes, unresponsiveness, tightly clenched jaws, asthma, rapid breathing, prolonged unconsciousness, and mental confusion upon waking. These symptoms indicate blood stasis that has become firm and immobile, making recovery difficult.

However, if the person is not in a state of mental confusion and suffers only from persistent pain and stasis, chest fullness, shortness of breath, and silence, but is still able to eat and drink a little when awake, the recommended treatment involves taking a modified version of "Su Zi Tao Ren Tang" with "Zhi Qiao" in the morning, and "Shu Xue Wan" in the evening. External treatment includes applying "Wan Ling Gao" and using a heated mixture of "Ding Tong San" for moxibustion or heat treatment, which may lead to recovery.

Additionally, it should be noted that any bifurcation in the bones throughout the body is also referred to as "Qi Gu." This is important information for students and practitioners of traditional medicine to be aware of.

The Manubrium

The "Bi Xin Gu (◇◇◇)" refers to the manubrium, also known as the "Jiu Wei Gu" or Pigeon Tail Bone. It is a fragile bone located between the Qi Gu (the junction of the clavicle bones) in the lower chest area. Injuries to this bone due to falls, impacts, or shocks result in persistent pain, a sensation of gas moving up and down the sides of the torso, abdominal pain, an inability to straighten the waist, and a tendency to hold the chest with both hands.

For such injuries, it is recommended to take "Ba Li San" internally. Externally, wash the area with a decoction of mugwort and vinegar, apply "Wan Ling Gao," and drink light yellow wine to quench thirst. It is advised to avoid tea, cold and raw foods, and porridge made from bran rice.

The Upper and Lower Lateral Ribs

The "Fu Gu(◇◇)" refers to the lower lateral ribs just beneath the chest. These ribs, two on each side, upper and lower, are prone to injury. The area above these ribs is protected by the elbow and arm, making it less susceptible to injury. The lower ribs near the abdomen are easier to treat because they can be grasped by hand, allowing for realignment in case of a fracture. A person with such an injury typically bows their head and stoops, experiences pain and moans, can only lie on their side and not on their back, and suffers from pain throughout the body when standing, as well as confusion, fainting, and a loss of appetite. Treatment involves taking "Zheng Gu Zi Jin Dan" internally, washing the area with "Ba Xian Xiao Yao Tang," applying "Wan Ling Gao," and using other medicines that disperse blood stasis to heal.

If the injury is to the second rib from the top, which may be broken or deeply bruised and collapsed, it is more challenging to treat due to its location above the diaphragm and difficulty in physically manipulating it. Even with forceful treatment, full recovery is difficult. Blood from the injury that remains on the diaphragm can form a cyst if it does not circulate properly with the aid of medication. Light cysts contain yellow fluid, while harder ones contain blood clots, potentially leading to chronic health issues.

The backbone

The back, from the large vertebrae at the lower part of the torso up to the waist, is commonly referred to as such. The bones here are known as the spinal bones or the vertebral column, and colloquially referred to as the backbone. This structure consists of a single column of twenty-one segments, extending from the end of the sacrum at the bottom to the shoulders at the top, supporting the internal organs. The bones on either side of the spine are attached in a horizontal overlapping fashion, curving forward to form the chest and ribs.

When affected first by exposure to cold and wind, and then by trauma from falls or blows, these areas can suffer from blood stasis and congealed knots. If the spinal tendons bulge and the bone joints are misaligned, a hunched back can develop. Treatment involves first massaging the tendons to soften them, then carefully aligning the bones back into place to straighten the back. Internally, "Zheng Gu Zi Jin Dan" is taken. Topically, "Ding Tong San" is applied, followed by a treatment with a heated iron tool to induce warmth before applying the medicine, and then "Hun Yuan Gao" is applied.

The Lumber Bones

The lumbar bones refer to the bones between the fourteenth, fifteenth, and sixteenth vertebrae of the spine. In cases of injury from falls or impacts, which lead to blood stasis and congealed knots, the individual is usually forced to lie face down, as lying on their back or side becomes impossible due to unbearable pain and stiffness in the lumbar muscles.

The recommended manual therapy involves aligning the spinal muscles inward towards the vertebral column. The practitioner, standing on an elevated surface, lifts the patient's hands high, which fully stretches the spinal muscles. Then, the patient is instructed to lie on their back and arch their chest, which straightens the vertebral column and alleviates the condition.

Internally, "Bu Jin Wan" (Tendon-Reinforcing Pills) should be taken. Externally, "Wan Ling Gao" (Myriad Spirit Ointment) should be applied, and "Zhi Tong San" (Pain-Relief Powder) should be used for moxibustion and ironing treatments.

Tailbone

The coccyx, also known as the tailbone, is characterized by its broad top and narrow bottom, and it supports the bones of the lower spine. On each side, it has four holes, collectively referred to as the "Eight Holes". The final segment of the coccyx is known as the "Tail Gate," also called the "End Bone," "Peg Bone," "Poverty Bone," or commonly as the "Tail Vertebra."

In cases where there is swelling or congestion due to sitting or squatting, which often extends to the lower back and hips, it is recommended to internally take "Zheng Gu Zi Jin Dan" (Bone-Setting Purple Gold Pills), wash the area with "Hai Tong Pi Tang" (Sea Tung Tree Bark Decoction), and apply "Wan Ling Gao" (Myriad Spirit Ointment).

Bones at the Four Limbs

SHOULDER BONES

The bone at the shoulder end, specifically the upper ridge of the bone socket of the shoulder swelling, contains the upper end of the humerus, situated at a point called the shoulder joint, where the shoulder blade and humerus meet, known as the shoulder head. Below, it attaches to the spine and back, forming a wing-like structure called the scapula.

If injured from a fall, the hand is likely to bend and turn backward, causing the bone seam to split open, making it impossible to lift or move forward, with the only movement being a twist behind the ribs. This leads to a congestion of qi (energy) and blood in the elbow, causing it to swell like a mallet. This swelling does not extend beyond the wrist, and both hands may experience tendon swelling and stagnation of blood. If the swollen area feels like being pricked by needles and doesn't move, it indicates that the blood will turn into pus, leading to the wrist and palm feeling cold or numb.

If the humerus protrudes, it should be pushed back into its socket and the tendons should be manipulated inward to reset the position of the elbow, arm, and wrist. For treatment, internal administration of "Bu Jin Wan" (Tendon-Strengthening Pills) is recommended, along with the application of "Wan Ling Gao" (Myriad Spirit Ointment). The affected area can be washed with "Hai Tong Pi Tang" (Sea Tung Tree Bark Decoction), and applications of "Bai Jiao Xiang San" (White Resin Powder), or the juice of "Jin Fei Cao" (Gold Boiling Herb) may also be beneficial.

The Humerus

The humerus is the bone located from below the shoulder to above the elbow. The arm, commonly referred to as the "arm" or "forearm," represents the two major limbs of the upper body. Injuries to the humerus can occur from various accidents such as falls from horses or carriages, leading to fractures, diagonal breaks, amputations, or shattering of the bone. A fracture caused by a blow may result in fragmented bones, whereas a fall-induced fracture usually does not produce bone fragments. Such injuries can cause swelling, pain, mental agitation, and a general feeling of numbness and coldness throughout the body.

Treatment involves manual techniques, aligning the tendons above, below, in front, and behind the injury to restore proper alignment. The injured bone seam is also massaged and adjusted to be straightened. A small fir board is then used to secure the area, wrapped externally with white cloth. Internally, "Zheng Gu Zi Jin Dan" (Bone-Setting Purple Gold Pill) should be taken, and "Wan Ling Gao" (Myriad Spirit Ointment) should be applied externally. If the swelling does not subside, an external wash with "San Yu He Shang Tang" (Bruise-Relieving and Injury-Harmonizing Decoction) should be used.

The Elbow Bone

The elbow bone is located at the joint where the upper and lower arm bones meet, commonly known as the "goose nose bone." In the event of a fall causing the tip of the elbow to protrude upward, resulting in unceasing pain and sweating with shivering, manual techniques should be used to flip the arm bone and pull the elbow bone so that it realigns properly. The slanted and bent tendons should be manually massaged and straightened. Although the elbow might be able to hang down or be raised immediately after the treatment, it is still best to focus on rest and recuperation. If there is swelling and pain, it is appropriate to take "Zheng Gu Zi Jin Dan" (Bone-Setting Purple Gold Pill) internally and apply "Wan Ling Gao" (Myriad Spirit Ointment) externally.

The Arm Bone

The arm bone, extending from the elbow to the wrist, consists of two parts: the main bone, which is larger and connects to the tip of the elbow, and the auxiliary bone, smaller and more slender, commonly known as the "wrap-around bone." These two bones are stacked and rely on each other, both connecting to the wrist bone. Arm bone injuries often occur due to fractures from impacts. Either both the main and auxiliary bones can be broken, or just one of them. These fractures lead to blood stasis, clotting, and pain. To treat this, the broken ends are manually aligned, "Wan Ling Gao" (Myriad Spirit Ointment) is applied, and the area is wrapped in a bamboo mat and tightly bound with cloth strips. After three days, the mat is opened to inspect the area. If any misalignment is felt upon pressing the injured site with a finger, the clotted area should be massaged again to realign the bones. The ointment is then reapplied, and the arm is rewrapped in the bamboo mat. "Zheng Gu Zi Jin Dan" (Bone-Setting Purple Gold Pill) should be taken every morning.

The Wrist Bone

The wrist bone, also known as the palm bone, is the base of the five fingers, sometimes referred to as the "congested bone" or colloquially as the "tiger bone." It consists of six small bones that form the wrist, which is not a single solid mass. These bones are connected at the base to the ends of the main and auxiliary bones of the arm. The outermost bone of the wrist is called the "high bone," also known as the "sharp bone" or "ankle bone," and colloquially as the "dragon bone." Its ability to flexibly bend up and down is why the wrist is named as such. Injuries to the wrist typically occur when falling off a horse or carriage and landing on the palm. If the hand lands with the fingers touching the ground and folding back onto the arm, the wrist bones will likely separate.

To treat a wrist injury, which usually involves swelling and pain, the method involves massaging the wrist with both hands. Internally, "Zheng Gu Zi Jin Dan" (Bone-Setting Purple Gold Pill) should be taken, and "Wan Ling Gao" (Myriad Spirit Ointment) should be applied externally. If the back of the hand is bent backwards towards the arm, gently roll the back of the hand forward with both hands to reposition it, then massage the tendons to ensure proper alignment. For such cases, take "Ren Shen Zi Jin Dan" (Ginseng Purple Gold Pill) internally and apply "Hun Yuan Gao" (Primordial Ointment) externally.

The Bones of the Five Fingers

The bones of the five fingers are called phalanges, which are the primary sections of each finger. If they are broken due to impact, all five fingers usually suffer together, leading to swelling and pain because their tendons are interconnected. While the external part of the palm and the back of the hand seem indistinct and continuous, internally, they are formed by the interconnected primary sections of each finger's bones.

If both the back and the palm of the hand are hard, swollen, hot, and painful, it is crucial to properly align the joints to prevent future complications. If not treated promptly, the congested blood in the area may later turn into pus. For those with robust energy, taking a medicine for treating boils and poison can lead to recovery; however, in those with weak energy, the condition may lead to persistent discharging wounds. The treatment involves washing the area with a decoction for dispersing blood stasis and healing injuries, and applying "Wan Ling Gao" (Myriad Spirit Ointment).

Finger Joint Bones

The "bamboo joint bone" refers to the intermediate phalanges of the fingers. In cases of injury due to falls or blows, when these bones are fractured and the tendons bent, the finger cannot be straightened. By manipulating the bent joint with the hand, the finger can be straightened out. The treatment involves washing the area with a decoction for dispersing blood stasis and healing injuries, and applying "Wan Ling Gao" (Myriad Spirit Ointment).

If the area under the fingernail accumulates toxic blood, the nail is likely to fall off. The regrowth of the nail often results in a shape that is different from the original. If the injury is to the third phalanx, the treatment is the same as for the intermediate phalanx. The nail on this phalanx is referred to as the claw nail.

The Hip Bone

The "hip bone," also known as the "iliofemoral bone" or "trochanter," is the bone that forms the hip. If one is predisposed to exposure to cold, damp winds and then suffers an injury from a fall or blow, blood stasis and clots can form, leading to swelling, hardness, and tendon inversion, making it difficult to walk straight. In cases where the tendons are shortened, the person may walk on tiptoes; if the bones are misaligned, the buttocks may protrude and cause an uneven gait.

The appropriate treatment involves manually manipulating and pressing the hip bone back into place, and repositioning the inverted tendons forward. This approach can effectively alleviate the condition. The patient should take "Jiawei Jianbu Huqian Pills" (modified vigorous step tiger hidden pills), use fumigation and wash with "Haitongpi Soup" (sea tongpi decoction), and apply moxibustion with "Ding Tong San" (pain fixing powder).

The Outer Concavity of the Hip Bone

The term "◈◈" (Huántiào) refers to the outer concavity of the hip bone, which is shaped like a socket designed to accommodate the upper end of the femur, resembling a pestle. This area is also known as the "◈" (Jī) or "◈◈" (Bǐshū), and is the location of the Huantiao acupoint. Injuries in this area can occur due to falls or accidents, such as getting caught in stirrups, leading to dislocation or misalignment of the joint, resulting in bruising, swelling, and pain, making it difficult to walk or causing an uneven, limping gait.

For treatment, it is recommended to first take "Zhenggu Zijin Dan" (bone-setting purple gold pills), wash the area with "Haitongpi Soup" (sea tongpi decoction), and apply "Wanling Ointment". Additionally, regularly taking "Jianbu Huqian Pills" (vigorous step tiger hidden pills) can be beneficial.

Thigh Bone

The "◇◇◇" (Dà jiàn gǔ), also known as the "◇◇" (Bǐ gǔ), refers to the femur or thigh bone. The upper end of this bone resembles a pestle and fits into the socket of the hip joint, known as the "◇◇" (Bǐshū), while the lower end is shaped like a hammer and is collectively referred to as the "◇" (Gǔ), denoting the major support of the lower body, commonly known as the thigh bone. Injuries to this bone, such as fractures and swelling due to a fall from a horse, can lead to symptoms like black and purple discoloration, a feeling of coolness, and the appearance of white blisters on the skin, indicating a severe injury where the bone is fractured and qi (vital energy) is depleted, making treatment challenging.

For younger individuals with ample energy and blood, even if there are symptoms of swelling and pain without unconsciousness or white blisters, treatment is possible. The method involves massaging the fractured bone with both hands, manipulating it back into place, and then pressing the injured area with fingers to ensure no misaligned bones. The area is then wrapped with a bamboo splint. "Zhenggu Zijin Dan" (bone-setting purple gold pills) should be taken every morning. After three days, the splint is removed to check for any unevenness, and if found, the tendons are twisted and smoothed out, followed by application of "Wanling Ointment" and re-wrapping with the bamboo splint.

Kneecap Bone

The "◇◇◇" (Xīgàigǔ), also known as the "◇◇" (Liánhái) or "◇◇" (Bìngǔ), refers to the patella or kneecap. It is round and flat, covering the ends of the femur and tibia. Tendons attach to its inner surface, extending from the thigh down to the foot's dorsum, passing over the bone.

Injuries to the knee, such as a blow or fall, can cause the kneecap to shift upwards, leading to swelling of its tendons and connected tendons inside. These inner tendons are linked to the waist and hips, often resulting in waist pain and difficulty bending. If the kneecap moves downwards, it can lead to swelling in the bone or a sensation of coldness and hardness in the feet, affecting walking and causing a dragging, skewed gait.

If the kneecap is dislocated outward, the inner tendons swell, while an inward dislocation results in straight tendon swelling. It's important to carefully examine the direction of the misalignment and use massage and manipulation techniques to reposition the bone. Internally, taking "Bǔjīn Wán" (Tendon-Strengthening Pills) and applying "Dìngtòng Sǎn" (Pain-Relieving Powder) with moxibustion can be beneficial. Fumigation with "Bāxiān Xiāoyáo Tāng" (Eight Immortals Carefree Decoction) can also promote healing.

Bones of the Lower Leg

The "◇◇◇" (Xiǎotuǐgǔ) refers to the bones of the lower leg, located between the knee and the ankle, commonly known as the "◇◇" (Jìnggǔ). There are two bones in this region: the one in front is called the "◇◇" (Chénggǔ), also known as the "◇" (Gǔ), which is thicker, and the one at the back is called the "◇◇" (Fǔgǔ), also commonly known as the "◇◇◇" (Láotánggǔ), which is thinner.

In cases of injury due to falls or blows, if the bone protrudes outwards, causing the flesh to tear and continuous bleeding, along with severe pain and moaning, reduced appetite, and especially if the individual is already weak in terms of energy and blood, the situation can become critical. The recommended treatment involves manually repositioning the bone by aligning the tendons and applying the "Wàn Líng Gāo" (Myriad Spirits Ointment). The leg should then be wrapped in bamboo splints and covered with white cloth. Initially, the "Zhènggǔ

Zǐjīn Dān" (Bone-Setting Purple Gold Pill) should be taken, followed by "Jiànbù Hǔqián Wán" (Tiger-Hiding Pills for Strengthening Steps).

The Ankle Bones

The "◇◇" (Huáigǔ) refers to the ankle bones, located below the lower leg bones and above the bones of the foot, characterized by two protrusions on each side. The inner protrusion is called the "◇◇" (Nèihuái), commonly known as the "◇◇" (Hégǔ), and the outer protrusion is the "◇◇" (Wàihuái), commonly referred to as the "◇◇" (Hégǔ).

Injuries such as falling from a horse or walking incorrectly can lead to conditions where the heel bone shifts forward, the toes point backward, and the tendons and flesh become swollen and painfully inflamed. The initial treatment involves manually adjusting the tendons and bones to their proper position. Then, the heel bone is stabilized using bamboo splints, fastened above the lower leg bones. After three days, the fastenings are removed to check the condition. A pillow is placed under the foot, and the tendons are gently supported and massaged, with particular attention to any knots in the tendons, ensuring they are smoothed out. Internally, the "Zhènggǔ Zǐjīn Dān" (Bone-Setting Purple Gold Pill) is administered, along with the application of moxibustion and "Dìng Tòng Sàn" (Pain-Setting Powder), and washing with "Hǎitóngpí Tāng" (Sea Tung Tree Bark Decoction). "Jiànbù Hǔqián Wán" (Tiger-Hiding Pills for Strengthening Steps) is also regularly taken.

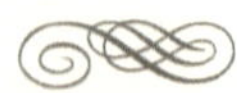

IF THERE IS SLIGHT improvement and then the patient engages in strenuous activities too soon, it can cause the end of the lower leg bone to twist inward, leading to a prominent and swollen inner ankle, or twist outward, causing the outer ankle to become prominent and swollen. This results in congested and coagulated blood vessels, weakened mobility, and an uneven footing, making treatment quite challenging.

Bones of the Foot Dorum

The "◇◇" (Fúgǔ) refers to the bones of the dorsum of the foot, also known as "◇◇" (Zúfū) or commonly called the top of the foot. These bones are essentially the base bones of the toes. Injuries to this area can occur from various causes, such as falls, being struck by heavy objects, or being crushed by vehicles or horses. If the injury is limited to the tendons and muscles, it is generally easier to treat; however, if the bones are damaged, treatment is often more challenging.

The initial treatment involves gently massaging the area by hand to help align the bones and relax the tendons. The injured area should be washed with decoctions such as "Hǎitóngpí Tāng" (Sea Tung Tree Bark Decoction) and "Bāxiān Xiāoyáo Tāng" (Eight Immortals Carefree Decoction), and "Wànlíng Gāo" (Myriad Spirits Ointment) should be applied. Internally, remedies that relax the tendons and alleviate pain should be taken, along with "Jiànbù Hǔqián Wán" (Tiger-Hiding Pills for Strengthening Steps) and "Bǔjīn Wán" (Tendon-Replenishing Pills).

Bone sof the Five Toes

The "◇◇◇◇" (Zú Wǔ Zhǐgǔ) refers to the bones of the five toes of the foot. "◇" (Zhǐ) means the toes of the foot, distinguishing them from the fingers of the hand, and they are commonly referred to as "foot joints." The number of joints in the toes is the same as in the fingers of the hand. The rounded, protruding bone on the inner side at the base of the big toe is known as "◇◇" (Hégǔ), also called "◇◇" (Gūguǎi) in common parlance.

Injuries to the toe bones are often similar to those of the "◇◇" (Fúgǔ), the bones of the top of the foot. However, injuries to the toes are more common due to running and hurried movements. The treatment methods for toe bone injuries are the same as those for the "◇◇."

Heel Bones

The "◇◇" (Gēngǔ) refers to the heel bone of the foot. It supports the ends of the two bones of the lower leg, and a large tendon, commonly known as the "foot cramp tendon," is attached to it. This tendon extends from the heel bone, passes over the ankle bone, reaches the inside of the calf, and goes up to the midsection. It then proceeds over the buttocks to the spine, up to the top of the head, and from the back of the brain forward to the eyes; all these areas are connected by this tendon.

Injuries such as falling off a horse or a misstep that cause the heel bone to twist forward and the toes to point backward can be severe. Even if the bone is not shattered but is dislocated, the tendons from the foot to the spine are affected, losing their normal tension and causing clenched, painful sensations. The appropriate treatment involves repositioning the bone to its original state and using medicinal remedies, following the same methods as previously mentioned.

Extended Discussion of Orthopedic Techniques

In modern orthopedics, which corresponds to the ancient practice of treating injuries from falls and trauma, the focus is on understanding blood conditions. It's essential first to distinguish whether there is blood stasis or excessive blood loss, and then apply appropriate internal treatment methods to avoid mistakes. In cases where the skin is not broken but there is internal damage, there is often blood stasis; whereas open wounds usually lead to excessive blood loss. The treatment for these two scenarios differs. For blood stasis, it's appropriate to use treatments that promote circulation and removal of stasis; for blood loss, nourishing and replenishing treatments are suitable. However, if there is neither much bleeding nor blood stasis, external treatment methods should be used.

Moreover, one must carefully assess the severity, depth, and location of the injury, as well as the differences in the meridians, qi, and blood. It's crucial to first eliminate blood stasis, harmonize the nutrients, and alleviate pain, and then nurture the qi and blood for effective healing. For injury cases and other complex conditions not fully covered here, they are categorized and detailed in subsequent sections, and students of this field should study them thoroughly.

Symptoms of internal injuries

IN CASES OF INJURIES from falls, trauma, or tumbling, if stagnant blood remains inside the body, regardless of the meridian involved, the liver is primarily affected. This is because the liver governs blood; hence, when bad blood coagulates and stagnates, it is attributed to the liver. Pain often occurs in the ribs, flanks, and lower abdomen, which are all areas along the liver meridian. If there is swelling, severe pain, fever, or spontaneous sweating, it is appropriate to carefully assess whether the condition is of excess or deficiency before using medicines that regulate blood and unblock the meridians.

The Qing physician Wang Haogu said: "In cases of injuries from falling from heights or collisions, where stagnant blood accumulates in the heart, abdomen, or chest and does not disperse, medicines should be applied according to the upper, middle, and lower Jiao (burners) of the body. For stagnation in the upper part, Rhino Horn and Rehmannia Decoction is appropriate; for the middle part, Peach Kernel Qi-Raising Decoction is suitable; and for the lower part, remedies like Di Dang Decoction are recommended."

"Huangdi Neijing" (Yellow Emperor's Inner Canon) states: "Injuries to the form cause pain, while injuries to the qi cause swelling." It also says: "If swelling occurs first followed by pain, it indicates an injury to the form and qi; if pain occurs first followed by swelling, it indicates an injury to the qi and form." In cases of injuries from falling, spraining, or twisting, or when anger causes qi stagnation and blood coagulation, as well as in cases of inherent weakness of the primary qi, injuries due to shouting or yelling, overconsumption of harsh medicines, or application of cold and cooling external remedies leading to qi and blood coagulation, all should be treated with remedies that invigorate the blood and regulate the qi.

Injuries with bleeding

IN CASES OF INJURIES with bleeding, either from the injured area or from various orifices, this condition is due to excessive liver fire and blood heat deviating from its proper pathways, resulting in reckless flow. Modified Xiao Yao San should be used to clear heat and nourish the blood. If the central qi is weak and the blood flows recklessly due to lack of adherence, use Modified Si Jun Zi Tang (Four Gentlemen Decoction) and Bu Zhong Yi Qi Tang (Tonify the Middle and Augment the Qi Decoction). If the primary qi internally collapses and cannot contain the blood, use Du Shen Tang (Solitary Ginseng Decoction) with added processed ginger to restore yang; if there is no response, urgently add aconite (Fu Zi). For blood stasis internally leading to vomiting of blood, use Si Wu Tang (Four Substances Decoction) with added Bupleurum (Chai Hu) and Scutellaria (Huang Qin). In cases of injury compounded by exertion, anger causing abdominal distension and discomfort, or overuse of cold and toxic medicines leading to damage of the yang meridians, this results in vomiting blood, nosebleed, blood in stool, or blood in urine; if the injury affects the yin meridians, it results in blood stasis, blood clots, and darkening of the muscles. These are all signs of organ deficiency and dysfunction of the meridian pathways. Urgent tonification of the spleen and lung organs is required for recovery.

Injury-induced blood stasis

THE CONDITION OF INJURY-induced blood stasis and widespread accumulation results from falls and stagnation of blood. This happens because when qi flows and disperses, blood follows and coagulates. It may accumulate in the limbs and joints, remain in the chest, abdomen, waist, or hips, or manifest as diffuse swelling or clots. Initially, these conditions are associated with stagnation of liver and spleen fire. Urgently use the scallion moxibustion method, and internally administer Xiao Chai Hu Tang to clear liver fire. Subsequently, use Ba Zhen Tang to strengthen the spleen and stomach, or Yi Qi Yang Rong Tang for long-term natural recovery. If there is ulceration and qi-blood deficiency over time, Shi Quan Da Bu Tang is appropriate; for ulceration with cold pathogenic stagnation that fails to heal, Dou Chi Bing (fermented soybean cake) should be used for dispersal. If qi and blood are not replenished, if care in daily life and emotional states is neglected, or if cold and reducing drugs are improperly used, these conditions are considered incurable.

Injuries with wwelling and pain

IN CASES OF INJURY with swelling and pain, the cause is often blood stasis and coagulation causing pain. If there is swelling accompanied by a sensation of heaviness, with the skin turning blue or black, and in severe cases fever, thirst, and sweating, this indicates obstruction in the meridians and channels, and injury to the yin blood. It is appropriate to first perform bloodletting to remove the stagnant blood and clear obstructions, followed by administering Si Wu Tang to regulate the condition.

Pain caused by blood deficiency

IN CASES OF INJURY where pain is caused by blood deficiency, the symptoms include fever, thirst, irritability, dizziness, and worsening in the late afternoon. This indicates a condition of yin deficiency with internal heat. The appropriate treatment is Ba Zhen Tang (Eight Treasure Decoction) with the addition of Dan Pi (Moutan Bark), Mai Dong (Ophiopogon), Wu Wei Zi (Schisandra), Rou Gui (Cinnamon Bark), and Gu Sui Bu (Drynaria) to address the condition.

Vomiting with black blood

IN CASES OF INJURY where there is vomiting of black blood, the initial cause is usually a fall or trauma, leading to damaged blood flowing into the stomach and epigastric region. The vomited blood is black in color, resembling soybean juice. For those with a robust physical constitution and strong energy, Bai He San (Lily Bulb Powder) is used. For those with a weaker constitution and energy, a modified version of Chuan Xiong Cha Tiao San (Ligusticum Chuanxiong Powder to be Taken with Green Tea) is recommended.

Injury with fever

IN CASES OF FEVER DUE to injury, if it is caused by excessive bleeding leading to a large and hollow pulse that disappears upon firm pressure, this is a fever due to blood deficiency. Dang Gui Bu Xue Tang (Angelica Blood-Nourishing Decoction) should be used. If the pulse is deep and faint, feeling soft and weak upon pressure, this indicates a fever due to excessive yin, and Si Jun Zi Tang (Four Gentlemen Decoction) with added processed ginger and aconite is appropriate. In cases of fever with restlessness and muscle twitching, this is due to loss of blood, and Sheng Yu Tang (Holy Healing Decoction) is recommended. If there is unceasing sweating along with the fever, this indicates hemorrhagic shock, for which Du Shen Tang (Single Ginseng Decoction) is suitable. In cases of hemorrhagic shock, those with a solid pulse are harder to treat, whereas those with a fine, small pulse are easier to treat.

Injury with muscle pain

IN CASES OF INJURY where there is muscle pain, it is caused by stagnation of the nutritive and defensive Qi. Fu Yuan Tong Qi San (Revive the Source and Unblock Qi Powder) should be used. When there is pain between the tendons and bones, it indicates damage to the Qi of the liver and kidneys, for which Liu Wei Di Huang Wan (Six-Ingredient Pill with Rehmannia) is recommended.

Injury with bone pain

IN CASES OF INJURY where there is bone pain, it indicates a minor injury. In cases of severe injury, where there is either a fracture or breakage, manual therapy is required, and the methods have been detailed in a previous section. In cases of minor injuries such as bumps and bruises causing pain between the bones, without any change in the color of the flesh, external application of the scallion ironing method and internal consumption of Myrrh Pills, along with the daytime use of Rehmannia Pills, will lead to recovery.

Injury with chest and abdominal pain

IN CASES OF INJURY presenting with chest and abdominal pain and discomfort, the cause is often due to actions such as jumping, beating the chest, twisting, lifting heavy weights, overexertion, or anger. If the chest and abdomen feel better when touched, it indicates liver fire injuring the spleen; in such cases, use Si Jun Zi Tang (Four Gentlemen Decoction) with the addition of Chai Hu (Bupleurum) and Shan Zhi Zi (Gardenia). If there is an aversion to being touched, it suggests blood stasis in the liver meridian; use Si Wu Tang (Four Substances Decoction) with added Chai Hu, Shan Zhi Zi, Tao Ren (Peach Kernel), and Hong Hua (Safflower). If there is discomfort and pain in the chest and ribs, fever, and afternoon fever, it indicates injury to the liver meridian's blood; use modified Xiao Yao San (Free and Easy Wanderer Powder).

If there is discomfort and pain in the chest and ribs, poor appetite, and reduced thoughtfulness, it signifies injury to the liver and spleen qi; use Si Jun Zi Tang with added Chuan Xiong (Szechuan Lovage), Dang Gui (Angelica), Chai Hu, Shan Zhi Zi, and Dan Pi (Moutan Bark). If there is bloating in the chest and abdomen, poor appetite, and reduced thoughtfulness, it suggests stagnation of liver and spleen qi; use Liu Jun Zi Tang (Six Gentlemen Decoction) with added Chai Hu, Chuan Xiong, and Dang Gui. If there is an obstruction in the chest and abdomen, poor appetite, and insomnia, it indicates stagnation of spleen qi; use modified Gui Pi Tang (Restore the Spleen Decoction). If there is phlegm and qi obstruction, stagnation of spleen and lung qi, use Er Chen Tang (Two-Cured Decoction) with added Bai Zhu (Atractylodes), Chuan Xiong, Dang Gui, Shan Zhi Zi, Da Ma

(Cannabis), and Gou Teng (Uncaria). If liver blood is injured due to the excessive use of wind-heat clearing herbs, resulting in intensified liver fire, or if the consumption of sugary alcohol leads to increased deficiency of kidney water and intensified spleen fire, or if the use of Da Huang (Rhubarb) and Shao Yao (Peony) internally injures the yin meridians, causing rectal bleeding, it can lead to chronic diseases in the young and strong, and in the elderly and weak, it often leads to an inability to recover.

Injury with swelling and pain in the ribs

IN CASES OF INJURY presenting with swelling and pain in the ribs, if the patient has normal bowel movements but experiences wheezing, coughing, and phlegm, it indicates liver fire encroaching on the lungs. Use Xiao Chai Hu Tang (Minor Bupleurum Decoction) with the addition of Qing Pi (Green Tangerine Peel) and Shan Zhi Zi (Gardenia) to clear it. If there is swelling and pain in the chest and abdomen, constipation, wheezing, coughing, and vomiting of blood, it is due to blood stasis and stagnation; use Dang Gui Dao Zhi San (Angelica Decoction for Guiding Out Stagnation) to relieve it.

"Huangdi Neijing" (Yellow Emperor's Inner Classic) states: "The liver stores blood, and the spleen governs blood. As the liver belongs to the wood element and wood overacts on earth, the spleen qi must be deficient." It is advisable to first clear the liver and nourish the blood, so the stagnant blood does not coagulate and stagnate. Next, strengthen the spleen and stomach to ensure the abundance of qi and blood. If aggressive and depleting methods are employed, those who are weak will become weaker, and stagnation will worsen, bringing swift misfortune.

Injury with abdominal pain

IN CASES OF INJURY presenting with abdominal pain, if there is constipation and severe pain upon pressing, it indicates internal blood stasis. Use modified Tiao Qi Tang (Regulating Qi Decoction) to purge it. If pain persists after purging and remains upon pressing, it means the blood stasis is not completely resolved. Use modified Si Wu Tang (Four-Substance Decoction) to nourish and mobilize the blood. If the abdomen hurts but feels better upon pressing, it's due to injury of the blood and qi; use Si Wu Tang with added Ginseng and Bai Zhu to nourish and harmonize. If there's pain in the chest and ribs after purging, it's due to liver blood injury; use Si Jun Zi Tang (Four Gentlemen Decoction) with Chuan Xiong and Dang Gui to nourish. If fever develops after purging, it indicates injury to the yin blood; use Si Wu Tang with Ginseng and Bai Zhu to nourish. If there's a chill after purging, it's due to yang qi injury; use Shi Quan Da Bu Tang (Ten Complete Great Tonifying Decoction) to nourish. If there's both chill and fever after purging, it's due to injury of both qi and blood; use Ba Zhen Tang (Eight Treasure Decoction) to nourish. If there's a desire to vomit after purging, it's due to stomach qi injury; use Liu Jun Zi Tang (Six Gentlemen Decoction) with Dang Gui to nourish. If diarrhea follows purging, it indicates injury to the spleen and kidneys; use Liu Jun Zi Tang with Rou Guo and Bu Gu Zhi to nourish. If hands and feet are cold, with confusion and sweating after purging, it's due to severe yang qi and cold deficiency; urgently use Shen Fu Tang. If there's coldness in the hands and feet, blue nails, and vomiting and diarrhea, it's an extreme case of spleen and kidney yang deficiency; urgently use a large dose of Shen Fu Tang. In cases of lockjaw, scattered hands, incontinence, heavy phlegm, blue lips, and cold body, these are signs of extreme deficiency and collapse; urgently use a large dose of Shen Fu Tang, which can often save lives.

Injury causing pain in the lower abdomen and the penis

IN CASES OF INJURY causing pain in the lower abdomen that radiates to the penis, it is due to stagnant blood and concurrent liver channel constraint and heat. It is appropriate to use Xiao Chai Hu Tang (Minor Bupleurum Decoction) with added Da Huang (Rhubarb), Huang Lian (Coptis), and Shan Zhi Zi (Gardenia). Once the pain stabilizes, follow up with a blood-nourishing formula for complete recovery. If this condition is mistakenly treated as a cold pattern and hot medicines are used, it can lead to serious danger in severe cases, or damage to the eyes in milder cases. Practitioners should be cautious in treatment.

Injury resulting in lower back or spinal pain

IN CASES OF INJURY resulting in lower back or spinal pain, which may be caused by falling or being struck, the pain is due to stagnant blood in the Bladder Meridian (Taiyang Channel). Di Long San (Earth Dragon Powder) is appropriate for treatment.

Injury with dizziness and vertigo

IN CASES OF INJURY with symptoms of dizziness and vertigo, this can be due to excessive use of aggressive treatments that harm the central Qi, leading to dizziness; or it can be due to excessive blood loss, also resulting in dizziness. If accompanied by abdominal bloating and vomiting, Liu Jun Zi Tang (Six-Gentleman Decoction) should be used. If there is also fever, thirst, and a lack of appetite, Shi Quan Da Bu Tang (Ten-Ingredient Tonic Decoction) is appropriate.

Injury with restlessness

IN CASES OF INJURY with symptoms of restlessness, flushed face, dry mouth, and thirst, if the pulse is large and feels almost absent when pressed, Dang Gui Bu Xue Tang (Angelica Blood-Tonifying Decoction) should be used. If restlessness is accompanied by spontaneous sweating and dizziness, Du Shen Tang (Solitary Ginseng Decoction) is appropriate. If there is restlessness and insomnia, Jia Wei Gui Pi Tang (Augmented Restore the Spleen Decoction) should be used. For restlessness with pain in the flanks, Chai Hu Si Wu Tang (Bupleurum and Four-Substance Decoction) is suitable. If the restlessness is due to excessive blood loss, Shen Yi Tang (Divine Healing Decoction) is recommended.

Injury with wheezing and coughing

IN CASES OF INJURY manifesting as wheezing and coughing, if it is due to excessive bleeding, resulting in a dark complexion, chest distension, pain in the chest and diaphragm, and wheezing, it indicates that qi deficiency has allowed blood to invade the lungs. In such cases, Er Wei Shen Su Yin (Two-Ingredient Ginseng and Perilla Drink) should be used urgently; delay can make it difficult to save the patient. If there is coughing up of blood, nosebleeds, and wheezing, it indicates that qi is rebelling and blood is congesting in the lungs. In this situation, it is only appropriate to activate blood circulation and move qi; purgative methods should not be used. Shi Wei Shen Su Yin (Ten-Ingredient Ginseng and Perilla Drink) is suitable for treatment.

Injury leading to stupor or unconsciousness

IN CASES OF INJURY leading to stupor or unconsciousness, where the patient is in a severe state of confusion and unaware of their surroundings, it is imperative to urgently administer Du Shen Tang (Solo

Ginseng Decoction). Even if there is internal blood stasis, purgatives must absolutely not be used. Instead, urgently use Hua Rui Shi San (Flower Pistil Powder) to internally transform the stasis. This is because purging is feared to lead to the loss of yin due to diarrhea. In cases where the primal qi (vital energy) is extremely weak, purgatives are especially contraindicated, and the aforementioned powder should be used for transformation.

For internal blood stasis with constipation, rhubarb and sodium sulfate (mirabilite) can be used. If the blood is congealed and does not move, it is necessary to use Muxiang (Aucklandia) and Rougui (Cinnamon Bark) in doses of two to three grams, mixed with hot wine for ingestion. This encourages the movement and discharge of blood, leading to recovery. For frail and weak individuals, when using sodium sulfate and rhubarb, it is essential to also add Muxiang and Rougui, cooked together. This approach uses the heat properties of these herbs to move the cold properties of the purgatives.

Injury causing vomiting

FOR CASES OF INJURY causing vomiting, the treatment depends on the underlying cause:

1. If the vomiting is due to severe pain or damage to the stomach caused by purgative treatments, use Si Jun Zi Tang (Four Gentlemen Decoction) with the addition of Dang Gui (Angelica Sinensis), Ban Xia (Pinellia), and fresh ginger.

1. If the vomiting is caused by anger resulting in liver damage, use Xiao Chai Hu Tang (Minor Bupleurum Decoction) with the addition of Shan Zhi Zi (Gardenia) and Fu Ling (Poria).

1. If the vomiting is due to excessive phlegm-heat, use Er Chen Tang (Two-Cured Decoction) with the addition of ginger-

fried Huang Lian (Coptis) and Shan Zhi Zi.

1. If the vomiting is due to weakness of the stomach qi, use Bu Zhong Yi Qi Tang (Tonify the Middle and Augment the Qi Decoction) with the addition of fresh ginger and Ban Xia.

1. If the vomiting is due to excessive blood loss, use Liu Jun Zi Tang (Six Gentlemen Decoction) with the addition of Dang Gui.

Injury resulting in thirst

FOR CASES OF INJURY resulting in thirst:

If the thirst is due to excessive blood loss, use Si Wu Tang (Four-Substance Decoction) with the addition of Ren Shen (Ginseng) and Bai Zhu (Atractylodes). If there is no response, use Ren Shen (Ginseng) and Huang Qi (Astragalus) to replenish qi, and Dang Gui (Angelica Sinensis) and Shu Di Huang (Processed Rehmannia) to nourish blood, or use Ba Zhen Tang (Eight-Treasure Decoction).

If the thirst is due to stomach heat damaging body fluids, use Zhu Ye Shi Gao Tang (Bamboo Leaf and Gypsum Decoction).

If the thirst is due to insufficient stomach fluids due to stomach weakness, use Bu Zhong Yi Qi Tang (Tonify the Middle and Augment the Qi Decoction).

If the thirst is due to excessive stomach fire, use Zhu Ye Shi Gao Tang (Bamboo Leaf and Gypsum Decoction).

If there is irritability and heat causing thirst, along with painful or difficult urination, it indicates kidney channel deficiency heat, which can only be remedied by Di Huang Wan (Rehmannia Pills).

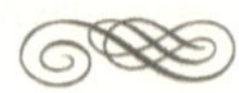

Injury with constipation

FOR CASES OF INJURY with constipation:

If constipation is due to blood deficiency and excessive fire in the large intestine, use Si Wu Tang (Four-Substance Decoction) with Run Chang Wan (Moisten Intestine Pill), or use pig bile to guide it.

If constipation is due to kidney deficiency and dryness, use Liu Wei Di Huang Wan (Six-Ingredient Pill with Rehmannia).

If constipation is due to deficiency of qi in the stomach and intestines, use Bu Zhong Yi Qi Tang (Tonify the Middle and Augment the Qi Decoction).

If there is constipation with firmness and pain in the abdomen, and strong interior qi, use Yu Zhu San (Jade Candle Powder).

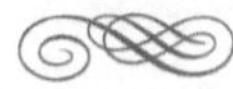

PLEASE NOTE that any practitioner who tries to apply these techniques and methods to treat their patients is advised to take proper training before the application. Readers of this book are advised to study TCM in greater details by reading my book "Every Person Is Their Own Best Doctor - Traditional Chinese Medicine In Practice."